IT All BEGINS WITH YOU

WORKBOOK

Janell Jones

Copyright © 2019 by Melanin Grace Publishing, LLC All rights reserved. No part of this publication may be reproduced, distributed or transmitted in any form or by any means, including photocopying, recording, or other electronic or mechanical methods, without the prior written permission of the publisher, except in the case of brief quotations embodied in critical reviews and certain other noncommercial uses permitted by copyright law. For permission requests, write to the publisher, addressed "Attention: Permissions Coordinator," at the address below.

Melanin Grace Publishing, LLC
P.O. Box 714
Pickerington, OH 43147
Website: http://janelljonesempowers.com
ISBN Paperback: 9781733643917

Disclaimer:

The information provided in this book is not a substitute for professional advice or therapy. The author makes no legal claims, and the material is not intended to replace the services of a certified professional.

Note From Author

I am excited that you are serious about taking control of your life by starting with YOU! Please be sure to complete the entire workbook. It is important to to be honest throughout the self-reflection process.

Sincerely,

Janell Jones

I take 100% responsibility for my life!

Know Yourself

Take the time to really get to know YOU!

The best way to get to know yourself is to spend time alone. Be intentional about spending 15 minutes alone with yourself today. Afterward, think about how it made you feel. Write your thoughts.

_____

_____

_____

_____

_____

_____

It is easy to get into the habit of saying yes to things, even those things we really don't want to do. Think about a time when you recently said yes to something, against your better judgment. How did it make you feel?

_____

_____

_____

_____

_____

_____

_____

It All Begins With You Workbook

Discover what you enjoy and what genuinely interests you. Take a moment to think about your talents and your interests. List them below.

_____

_____

_____

_____

_____

_____

_____

_____

Don't compare yourself to others. Your journey is your own. Write an affirmation to remind yourself that you are unique and your lane, destination, and appointed time are tailored for you and only you.

_____

_____

_____

_____

_____

_____

_____

_____

_____

It All Begins With You Workbook

Take the 16 Personalities test. What is your personality type? Do you think this is accurate? Was there anything that surprised you about your personality type? What are your overall thoughts about it? https://www.16personalities.com/free-personality-test

_____
_____
_____
_____
_____
_____
_____
_____

Now that you have completed the personality test, think about your purpose. How does the personality test connect with your purpose? Do they align?

_____
_____
_____
_____
_____
_____
_____
_____

I Am Enough!

Forgive Yourself

Learning to forgive will help you unblock your dreams. If you don't feel comfortable, move on to the next section.

Get out of denial. Be honest about your mistakes, especially the ones you are still holding on to. What mistake(s) from your past are you allowing to impact your life today?

_____

_____

_____

_____

_____

_____

_____

Think about the mistake you just reflected upon. Take a moment to truly acknowledge and take responsibility for it. How does this make you feel?

_____

_____

_____

_____

_____

_____

_____

_____

Now it's time to let it go. Engage in a physical exercise to demonstrate that you are letting it go. One way to do this is to write a letter about what happened and then bury the letter.

_____

_____

_____

_____

_____

_____

_____

_____

Be careful from whom you seek advice. Sometimes too many opinions can cloud your judgment. Think about your support network. List one or two people with whom you can safely share your feelings.

_____

_____

_____

_____

_____

_____

_____

_____

It All Begins With You Workbook

Now that you have forgiven yourself, don't look back. What steps are you going to take to focus on your windshield instead your rearview?

_____
_____
_____
_____
_____
_____
_____
_____
_____
_____
_____
_____
_____
_____
_____
_____
_____
_____
_____
_____
_____
_____
_____

It All Begins With You Workbook

Write yourself a forgiveness letter.

_____
_____
_____
_____
_____
_____
_____
_____
_____
_____
_____
_____
_____
_____
_____
_____
_____
_____
_____
_____
_____
_____
_____
_____
_____
_____

It All Begins With You Workbook

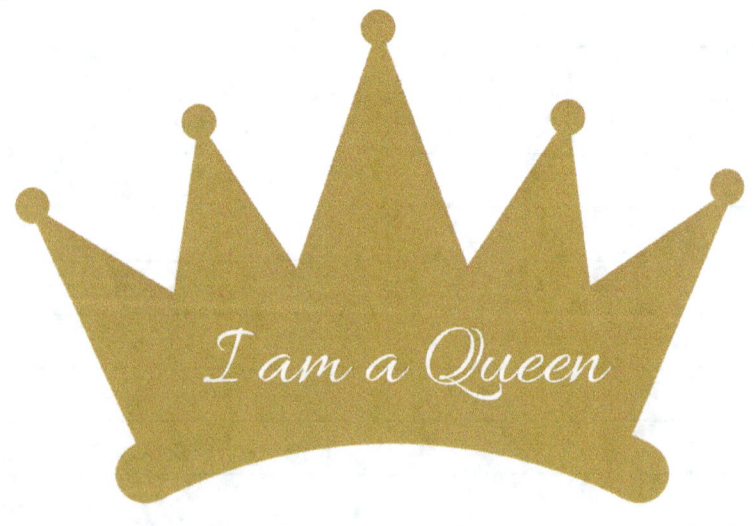

Release Yourself
(from pain)

You will learn how to release yourself from pain.

Acknowledge the pain. You cannot be free from what you will not admit. What are the sources of pain in your life that you need to acknowledge?

_____

_____

_____

_____

_____

_____

_____

Accept your feelings. You are always entitled to feel however it is that you feel. Do you make it a priority to stay in tune with your feelings? In what ways do you accept and own your feelings?

_____

_____

_____

_____

_____

_____

_____

_____

For many people, connecting to their spiritual source is helpful in releasing pain. One way to do that is through prayer. Write out your own personal prayer of healing.

_____
_____
_____
_____
_____
_____
_____
_____
_____

Now that you have acknowledged your pain, accepted your feelings, decided to heal, and connected to your spiritual source, it is time to RELEASE the pain. Write two ways that you will be intentional about releasing the pain.

_____
_____
_____
_____
_____
_____
_____
_____
_____

It All Begins With You Workbook

In what ways can you turn your pain into purpose?

___

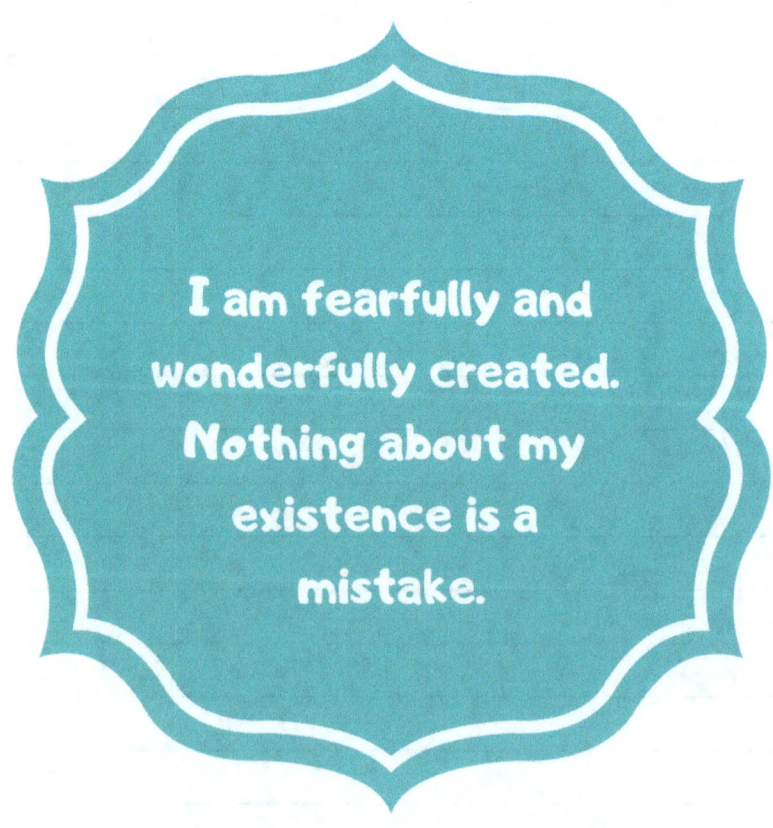

Love Yourself

Loving yourself is the foundation for every aspect of your life.

Own who you are. You can do this by accepting yourself as you are. What are some things about yourself that are easy for you to accept? What are some that are harder for you to accept?

_____
_____
_____
_____
_____
_____
_____
_____

Believe that you are worthy of love. Write an affirming statement indicating that you believe you are worthy of love. Include your name in your affirmation.

_____
_____
_____
_____
_____
_____

Be thankful for your uniqueness. Write down the things about yourself which you are thankful. Example: I am thankful for my generous heart.

_____

_____

_____

_____

_____

_____

_____

_____

_____

Celebrate yourself. Write five ways you can celebrate yourself.

_____

_____

_____

_____

_____

_____

_____

_____

_____

It All Begins With You Workbook

Write three love affirmations to say to yourself daily. Example: I love myself. I am the love of my life.

It All Begins With You Workbook

For the next three days, use the love affirmations that you created to affirm yourself. Each morning and evening state your love affirmations. Note your feelings.

Girl, You Got This!

Be Yourself

Walk in your authenticity.

Assess Yourself! Do you have trouble being yourself? If so, list the who, when, where and/or circumstance that prevents you from being comfortable with being your authentic self.

_____
_____
_____
_____
_____
_____
_____
_____

Do you have any fears around being your authentic self? What are they? Confess those fears so that you can conquer them. Know that you are fearfully and wonderfully made and there is no one like you.

_____
_____
_____
_____
_____
_____
_____
_____

It All Begins With You Workbook

List three ways you will work on building confidence in yourself.

_____
_____
_____
_____
_____
_____
_____
_____

List five ways to show up big and not play small.

_____
_____
_____
_____
_____
_____
_____
_____
_____
_____

It All Begins With You Workbook

Practice your confidence in the mirror or with a friend. How did it make you feel?

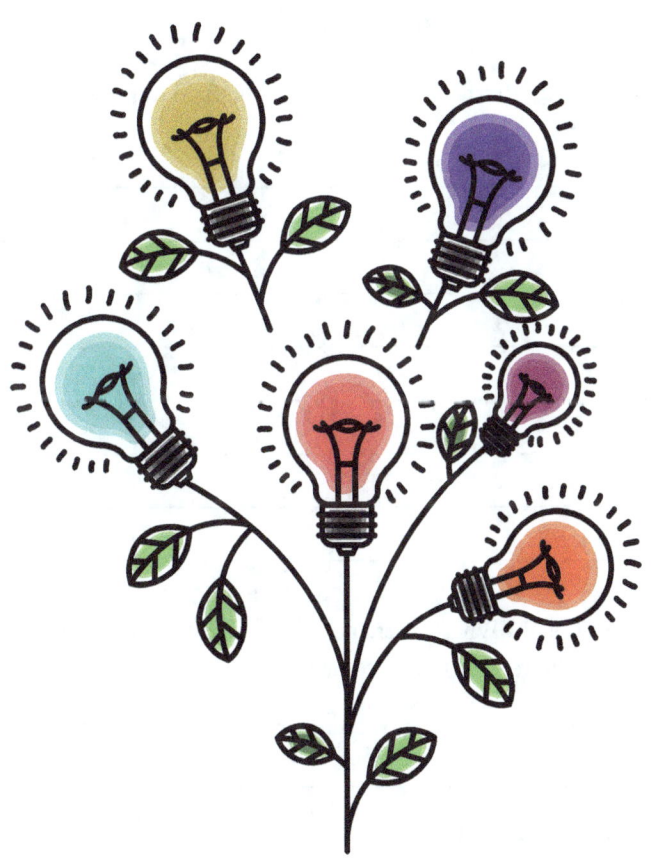

Promote Yourself

Shift your mindset.

Practice positive thinking. List ways you can shift your mind from negative thinking to positive thinking.

_____

_____

_____

_____

_____

_____

_____

Believe you are enough. What experiences have taught you that you are not enough? How are you working to overcome that?

_____

_____

_____

_____

_____

_____

_____

_____

_____

It All Begins With You Workbook

It is hard to maintain a positive mindset when you are surrounded by negativity. Make a list of negative people and/or things that you need to remove from your life.

_____
_____
_____
_____
_____
_____
_____
_____
_____
_____
_____
_____
_____
_____
_____
_____
_____
_____
_____
_____
_____
_____
_____

What standards do you have for yourself? In what ways do you need to shift them to get to the next level?

___

Because...
I'm Worth It!

Visualize Yourself

Success manifests from your thoughts.

What is it that you desire for yourself? Make a list of things that you desire. Be sure to be specific.

_____
_____
_____
_____
_____
_____
_____
_____
_____
_____
_____
_____
_____
_____
_____
_____
_____
_____
_____

It All Begins With You Workbook

Complete visualization exercise: Visualize your goals. Close your eyes, what do you see? How does it feel to visualize your goals?

_____
_____
_____
_____
_____
_____
_____
_____
_____
_____
_____
_____
_____
_____
_____
_____
_____
_____
_____
_____
_____
_____
_____

Complete a vision board
Tools:

- Poster board
- Scissors
- Glue
- Decorations (glitter, stickers)
- Magazines
- Pictures
- Whatever you like

Instructions:

Use the previous exercises to symbolize your vision with pictures or words. Be intentional with your vision. Don't just place pictures on the board. You can also complete a digital board using Canva (www.canva.com). This way you can have access to your board anytime.

It All Begins With You Workbook

Journaling is one way to stay on track toward meeting your goals. Get 3-5 journals and write your thoughts in them. Separate your journals by projects. Each journal should represent an individual project. What will you title each journal?

_____

_____

_____

_____

_____

_____

_____

_____

Take 10 minutes at the beginning and end of each day to meditate on your vision.

_____

_____

_____

_____

_____

_____

_____

_____

_____

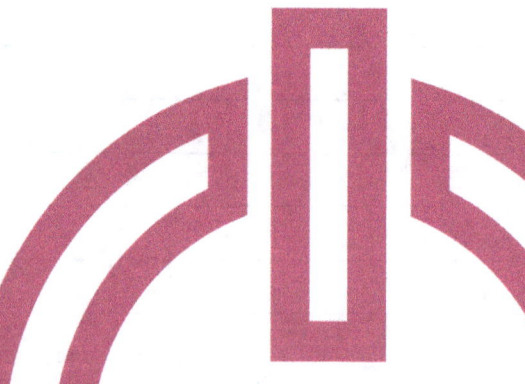

I am powerful. I have the ability to move mountains with my faith. I simply believe.

Apply Yourself

Now, put those thoughts into action!

What has held you back from reaching your dreams previously? Be honest.

_____

_____

_____

_____

_____

_____

_____

_____

As you think of taking actions to reach your dreams, what fears arise? List them and write counteractions for each fear.

_____

_____

_____

_____

_____

_____

_____

_____

_____

List 3-5 overarching goals you wish to complete.

_____
_____
_____
_____
_____
_____
_____
_____
_____

Create an action plan for each goal (worksheet on next page). Put dates for each overarching goal and action plan.

_____
_____
_____
_____
_____
_____
_____
_____
_____

Goal Attainment Worksheet

Overarching Goal _____

Completion date _____

Action steps

1. _____ Completion date _____
2. _____ Completion date _____
3. _____ Completion date _____
4. _____ Completion date _____
5. _____ Completion date _____

• •

Overarching Goal _____

Completion date _____

Action steps

1. _____ Completion date _____
2. _____ Completion date _____
3. _____ Completion date _____
4. _____ Completion date _____
5. _____ Completion date _____

Overarching Goal _____

Completion date _____

Action steps

1. _____ Completion date _____

2. _____ Completion date _____

3. _____ Completion date _____

4. _____ Completion date _____

5. _____ Completion date _____

• •

Overarching Goal _____

Completion date _____

Action steps

1. _____ Completion date _____

2. _____ Completion date _____

3. _____ Completion date _____

4. _____ Completion date _____

5. _____ Completion date _____

It All Begins With You Workbook

Overarching Goal _____

Completion date _____

Action steps

1. _____ Completion date _____

2. _____ Completion date _____

3. _____ Completion date _____

4. _____ Completion date _____

5. _____ Completion date _____

• •

Overarching Goal _____

Completion date _____

Action steps

1. _____ Completion date _____

2. _____ Completion date _____

3. _____ Completion date _____

4. _____ Completion date _____

5. _____ Completion date _____

Who are the people in your life who can help you achieve your goals? Make a list of people who celebrate you and want to see you successful.

_____

_____

_____

_____

_____

_____

_____

_____

List five ways you can invest in yourself. This may include courses, coaching, or mentorship. Always be sure to do research before spending money.

_____

_____

_____

_____

_____

_____

_____

_____

_____

It All Begins With You Workbook

Create 1-3 goals each morning or during lunch from your list of action steps (you may have to break them down even further). Take 30 minutes to an hour in the evening (or a time that is convenient) to complete each goal if you didn't complete a goal, roll them over to the next day.

_____
_____
_____
_____
_____
_____
_____
_____
_____
_____
_____
_____
_____
_____
_____
_____
_____
_____
_____
_____

enjoy every moment.

Care For Yourself

You need to be cared for too!

List five ways you will reward yourself.

_____
_____
_____
_____
_____
_____
_____
_____

What are some ways you can take care of your health?

_____
_____
_____
_____
_____
_____
_____
_____
_____
_____
_____

Create a list of boundaries that apply to five areas of your life: finances, personal time, relationships (family, friends, etc.), employment/entrepreneur, and self-care.

It All Begins With You Workbook

Think of toxic environments in your life. How will you eliminate them from your life and/or manage them until you can eliminate them?

_____
_____
_____
_____
_____
_____
_____
_____
_____
_____
_____
_____
_____
_____
_____
_____
_____
_____
_____
_____
_____
_____
_____
_____

It All Begins With You Workbook

Never feel guilty about caring for yourself. Self-care is essential. Write 3-5 self-care statements. Example: I deserve to care for myself.

_____

_____

_____

_____

_____

_____

_____

_____

_____

_____

_____

_____

_____

_____

_____

_____

_____

_____

_____

_____

_____

_____

_____

I am Thankful!

30-Day Gratitude Journal

For the next 30 days, write what you are grateful for. This will allow you to focus your energy on the positive. Set aside time to write in your journal daily. Reflect on your day and separate the positive from the negative.

Day 1

Month _____ Day _____ Year_____

_____
_____
_____
_____
_____
_____
_____
_____
_____
_____
_____
_____
_____
_____
_____
_____
_____
_____
_____

It All Begins With You Workbook

Day 2

Month _____ Day _____ Year_____

Day 3

Month _____ Day _____ Year_____

It All Begins With You Workbook

Day 4

Month _____ Day _____ Year_____

It All Begins With You Workbook

Day 5

Month _____ Day _____ Year_____

It All Begins With You Workbook

Day 6

Month _____ Day _____ Year_____

It All Begins With You Workbook

Day 7

Month _____ Day _____ Year_____

It All Begins With You Workbook

Day 8

Month _____ Day _____ Year _____

It All Begins With You Workbook

Day 9

Month _____ Day _____ Year_____

It All Begins With You Workbook

Day 10

Month _____ Day _____ Year_____

It All Begins With You Workbook

Day 11

Month _____ Day _____ Year_____

It All Begins With You Workbook

Day 12

Month _____ Day _____ Year_____

It All Begins With You Workbook

Day 13

Month _____ Day _____ Year _____

It All Begins With You Workbook

Day 14

Month _____ Day _____ Year_____

Day 15

Month _____ Day _____ Year_____

It All Begins With You Workbook

Day 16

Month _____ Day _____ Year_____

It All Begins With You Workbook

Day 17

Month _____ Day _____ Year_____

It All Begins With You Workbook

Day 18

Month _____ Day _____ Year_____

It All Begins With You Workbook

Day 19

Month _____ Day _____ Year_____

It All Begins With You Workbook

Day 20

Month _____ Day _____ Year _____

It All Begins With You Workbook

Day 21

Month _____ Day _____ Year_____

It All Begins With You Workbook

Day 22

Month _____ Day _____ Year_____

It All Begins With You Workbook

Day 23

Month _____ Day _____ Year_____

Day 24

Month _____ Day _____ Year_____

It All Begins With You Workbook

Day 25

Month _____ Day _____ Year_____

It All Begins With You Workbook

Day 26

Month _____ Day _____ Year_____

It All Begins With You Workbook

Day 27

Month _____ Day _____ Year_____

It All Begins With You Workbook

Day 28

Month _____ Day _____ Year_____

It All Begins With You Workbook

Day 29

Month _____ Day _____ Year_____

It All Begins With You Workbook

Day 30

Month _____ Day _____ Year_____

I Am Destined for Greatness!

About the Author

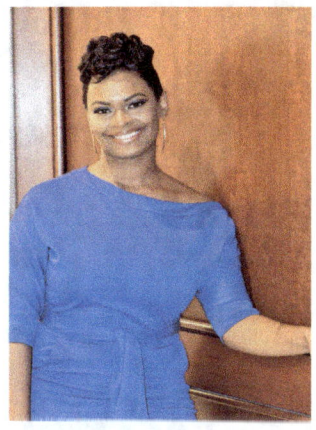

Janell Jones is on a journey to help women and girls to understand how important it is to love and know themselves. Janell's focus is to help others who feel unworthy, undervalue and unappreciated shift their mindset, take responsibility for their lives, and positively affirmed themselves.

Janell is a certified life coach, public speaker, business owner and author. She has an associates degree in psychology, bachelor's and a Master's degrees in Social worker. She is a licensed social worker.

It All Begins With You Workbook

For additional resources, please add *It All Begins With You* to your library.

Visit: http://bit.ly/janelljonesempowerscourses for the on-line course.

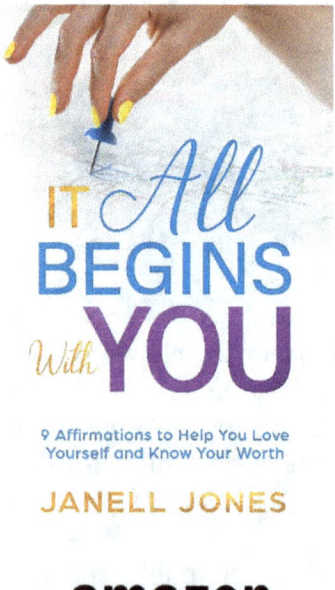

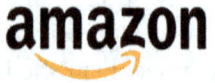

BARNES & NOBLE

www.ingramcontent.com/pod-product-compliance
Lightning Source LLC
Chambersburg PA
CBHW071221070526
44584CB00019B/3097